Gotta Minute?
Yoga
for
Health,
Relaxation & Well-being

Nirvair Singh Khalsa

Robert D. Reed Publishers
750 La Playa Street, Suite 647
San Francisco, CA 94121
Phone: 650/994-6570 • Fax: -6579
E-mail: 4bobreed@msn.com
http://www.rdrpublishers.com

Photography, Book Design and Layout
by Nirvair Kaur Khalsa
Editing and Typesetting by Nirvair Kaur Khalsa
and Pamela D. Jacobs, M.A.
Book Cover by Julia A. Gaskill at Graphics Plus

ISBN 1-885003-64-1

Library of Congress No. 00-105835

Produced and Printed in the United States of America

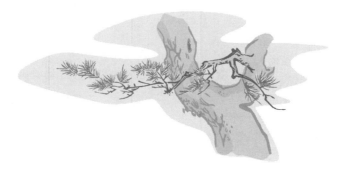

DEDICATION

With special love, devotion & reverence to
Yogi Bhajan, the Master of Kundalini Yoga,
without whom these teachings and myself as teacher
would not be possible.
Also my ongoing thanks & respect to the
Kundalini Research Institute and the
International Kundalini Yoga Teachers Association

Special Thanks To My Family...

Love and thanks to my wife and partner Nirvair Kaur Khalsa
for the photography, book design and her
continued vision of what is real and beautiful.
Hugs and thanks to my children, Siri Pritam Bhagvati Kaur
Khalsa and Har Rai Singh Khalsa for demonstrating the yoga
and being the wonderful, sophisticated souls
that they are.

NOTE TO READERS

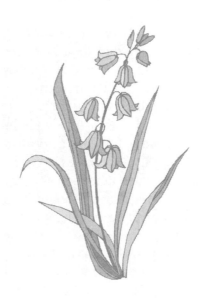

FOREWORD

I have known Nirvair for what seems like lifetimes and I am delighted to see this new book be published. I recommend his books and many videos to all of our students at Golden Bridge Nite Moon, a yoga center in Los Angeles.

Like his videos, _Yoga for Health, Relaxation and Well-being_ is very accessible to all people. There is a peaceful, universal and very practical quality to this book. I know you will enjoy and learn so much to make your lives more healthy and happy.

As a teacher and author of Kundalini Yoga books and videos, I have always fostered a comfortable, relaxed, and fun way of being in my classes. Yoga is about practice, but it is also about connection to our higher selves and connection to each other as human beings. Nirvair's new book has that power to help you make that connection. I urge you to practice these simple techniques and then share them with your friends and family.

Kundalini Yoga and Meditation will change your life for the better and quickly! It has helped so many people in countless ways. Blessings to you with the Universal Love of the Divine on your journey,

Gurmukh
Golden Bridge Nite Moon Yoga Center
Los Angeles. CA

Author of _Eight Human Talents_ (Harper/Collins)

Gotta Minute?
Yoga for Health, Relaxation and Well-being

TABLE OF CONTENTS

CHAPTER ONE - EXERCISES

CHAPTER TWO - BASIC BREATHS

CHAPTER THREE - HEAL YOUR BACK NOW!

CHAPTER FOUR - MEDITATIONS

CHAPTER FIVE - DEEP RELAXATION

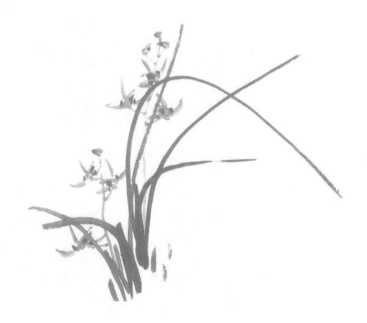

Introduction

Thank you for picking this book on Kundalini Yoga as taught by Yogi Bhajan. You are in for some wonderful experiences and pleasant surprises that relate to you own self discovery through the practice of the ageless science and art of Kundalini Yoga. You will find that the exercises, breaths and meditations in this book are very effective, although they take very little time. The "Heal Your Back Now!" series of exercises have helped thousands of people maintain a healthy back.

Kundalini Yoga by definition is an ancient and synergistic form of yoga practiced for centuries in India and the East. It incorporates the physical, mental and spiritual aspects of yoga into a cohesive and integrated system. Much of Kundalini Yoga was kept secret until Yogi Bhajan first came to America to teach it in 1969. It is dynamic in its' practice, vast in practical information and powerful in its' experience. It is perfect for people who want both the immediate and long-term benefits of yoga and a relaxed and uplifting experience of consciousness.

The techniques in this book take very little time and are well worth the investment. If you ever have the opportunity, take a class by a certified Kundalini Yoga instructor. If you do not have an instructor in your area you can go to my web site http://www.KundaliniYoga.net and buy a video for your home practice. In a class or a video on Kundalini Yoga, you will learn and practice physical postures, breathing exercises, stress release and relaxation techniques, guided imagery and affirmations, mantras, kriyas, and meditations. The benefits will be enhanced health and well being, greater physical flexibility, a more comfortable back, stronger and balanced immune, digestive, eliminative, and nervous systems. You will gain greater calmness, clarity, creativity, and improved concentration, a working understanding of the mind/body connection and a self-guided ability to relax and rejuvenate the mind, body and spirit. Learning and practicing yoga can serve you for your entire life. It is a life time skill that can be practiced at any age.

I have been teaching Kundalini Yoga at the University of Alaska Anchorage since 1975. There are several comments that I regularly get from students about these classes at the end of the session. Students find that they have a more comfortable back and spine. They are feeling more relaxed and better able to handle stress and generally have more positive sense of self and well being. The techniques in this book address these common challenges to daily life.

This reflects my experience of Kundalini Yoga as well. I have been practicing since 1969 and have found that the rewards of a regular practice are profound. Yoga treats the person as a whole creature; mind, body, emotions and spirit are positively affected and uplifted. Yoga is not a religion but provides a very firm foundation on all levels of being so that an individual may excel in any area of life.

In Kundalini Yoga we strive for balance in our practice. This means that while you exercise, it is good to gently challenge yourself, but not to overdo it. It is always fine to shorten the duration of an exercise. You can also modify an exercise to your special needs by changing the range of motion or even by sitting out an exercise altogether. If you are pregnant (usually it is OK to do anything in yoga for the first trimester) check with your midwife or doctor about what you can and cannot do in yoga.

You will have to modify exercises as your size increases. If you are overweight or have high blood pressure, have pre-existing injuries, it is always best to allow your doctor to advise you as to what you can and cannot do in yoga.

The "Healthy People 2010 Objectives" call for increases in physical flexibility increases in strength and endurance and a reduction in stress. Your participation with the techniques in this book will go along way to reach these objectives. I hope you enjoy these techniques and all the healthful and relaxing aspects of Kundalini Yoga.

Chapter 1

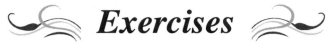

Exercises

Exercise Overview

Exercises in Yoga are called postures or asanas. Historically, Yoga was developed over a long period of time. It was developed by people experimenting with movements and with the angles that the body makes in certain positions. Humans are natural mimics so the yogis would copy the natural position or movement of an animal that they would observe in their environment. This is the reason that the common names of the exercises may relate to an animal like cow, cat or cobra.

When I recorded my first Yoga video in 1990, I sent a copy to the Library of Congress for a copyright. They immediately sent it back informing me that one cannot copyright human movements. This, of course, makes sense. Otherwise, if you could copyright a movement, you might have to pay someone every time you would scratch or blow your nose! You can copyright the order of movements so I sent the corrected application back and received my copyright. This anecdote illustrates a point that I love to make to students; yoga exercises were developed by human beings for human beings. They are natural, easy and fun.

These exercises can be practiced any time and anywhere that it is convenient to you. Exercises like the Shoulder Rolls and Neck Turns are terrific when you are sitting at your desk. Exercises like the Front Stretch and Basic Spine Flex can be practiced while you are watch television. You can just plop down on the floor and stretch while you watch. Definitely teach your children or grandchildren Lion Face! It brings out the child in everyone.

Yoga is best practiced in a series of exercises. This way the exercises can supplement and compliment each other for a synergistic affect. Truly, the sum is greater than the individual parts. The "Heal Your Back Now!" series is wonderful for the back and takes several of the individual exercises in this book and combines them together. While you practice this series be very aware of how your body feels and how it changes during the exercises. This self -awareness will grow and serve very well in every day life.

Please remember that we always strive for balance in our practice. This means that when you do any of these exercises, it is good to gently challenge yourself, but not to overdo it. It is always fine to shorten the duration of an exercise. You can also modify an exercise to your special needs by changing the range of motion.

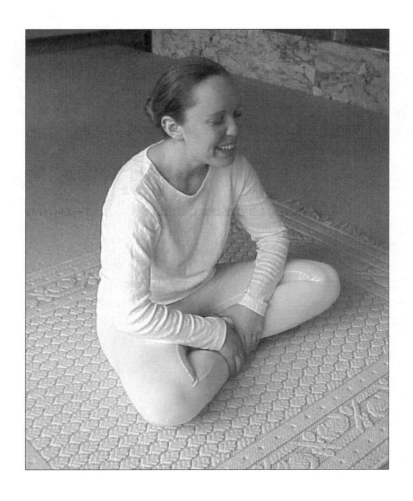

Basic Spine Flex for Lower Back

Time

One to five minutes.

Physical Position

Sit comfortably cross-legged tailor fashion. Have the hands on the shins right above the ankles.

Instruction

Inhale through the nose as you lift the chest up high and arch the lower back. As you exhale through the nose, slump back, tilting the pelvis, pushing the lower back out and letting the chest collapse. Keep the chin level to the ground and the shoulders down and relaxed throughout the exercise.

Comments

It stretches and strengthens the lower back. It changes brain wave patterns after three minutes to make you calm. Please remember that we always strive for balance in our practice. This means that when you do this exercise, it is good to gently challenge yourself, but not to overdo it. It is always fine to shorten the duration of an exercise. You can also modify an exercise to your special needs by changing the range of motion.

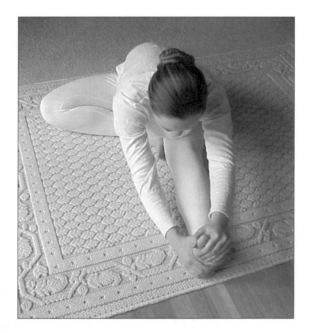

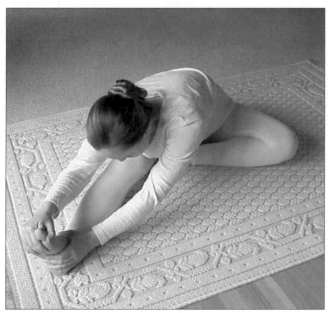

Front Stretch for Spine & Sciatic Nerve

Time

One to five minutes on each side.

Physical Position

Sit comfortably with the legs extended out in front of you straight.

Instruction

Stretch the left leg out in front of you straight; right foot against the inner thigh of the left leg, heel close to the groin. Tilt the pelvis forward and reach and catch on to the shin or foot with both hands. Gently stretch forward then down. Keep the chin at a right angle to the chest. Hold the position without bouncing. Use Long Slow Deep Breathing. Switch sides so that the right leg is extended and the left foot is against the inner thigh of the right leg. Hold the position without bouncing. Long Slow Deep Breathing.

Comments

It stretches the life nerve also known as the sciatic nerve. It is good for the lower back, stretches the hamstrings, and relaxes the quads. Please remember that we always strive for balance in our practice. This means that when you do this exercise, it is good to gently challenge yourself, but not to overdo it. It is always fine to shorten the duration of an exercise. You can also modify an exercise to your special needs by changing the range of motion.

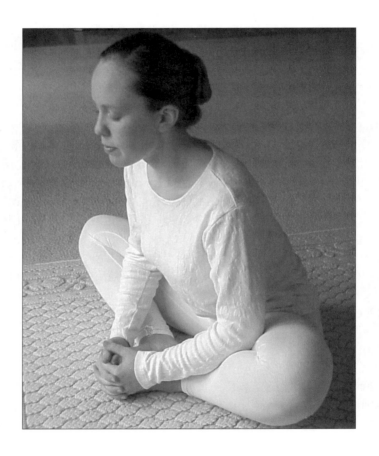

Butterfly Stretch for Hips

Time

One to five minutes.

Physical Position

Sit comfortably with the soles of the feet together.

Instruction

Hold on to the feet with hands, lean forward keeping the back straight and the chin at a 90° angle to the chest. Hold the position without bouncing. Use Long Slow Deep Breathing.

Comments

This exercise opens up and stretches the hips. It stretches the inner thigh and lower back. Please remember that we always strive for balance in our practice. This means that when you do this exercise, it is good to gently challenge yourself, but not to overdo it. It is always fine to shorten the duration of an exercise. You can also modify an exercise to your special needs by changing the range of motion.

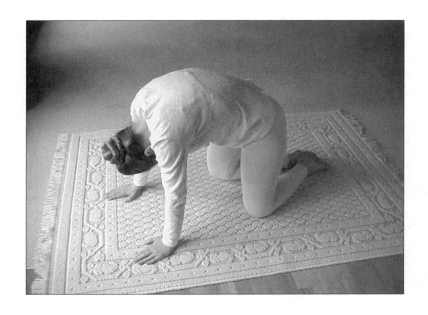

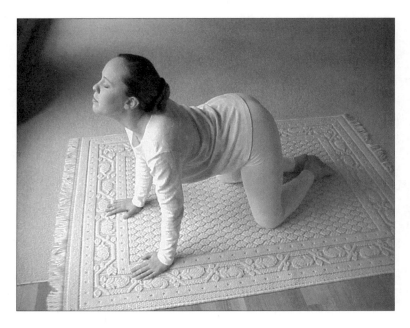

Cow/Cat Exercise for Total Spine

Time

One to three minutes.

Physical Position

The hands are straight down from the shoulders with the fingers pointing forward and the elbows locked straight. If your wrists bother you, then make your hands into fists, and place the knuckles on the ground. The knees are straight down from the hips and are separated by about six inches. Toes are uncurled.

Instruction

This is a two-part motion. You are going to inhale and tilt the pelvis forward in cow position and lift the head up and back. Now exhale, tilt the pelvis the opposite way and at the same time push up through the shoulders in cat position and bring the chin to the chest. Get the full range of motion with the head and neck. Inhale through the nose into cow, and exhale through the nose into cat. Continue. Make the motion very smooth in transition. When you have reached your full range of motion in one position then initiate the other position.

Comments

It is a total spine exercise. It brings extra circulation into the face and head. It releases stored energy for healing the body. It stimulates the higher glands in particular thyroid, pituitary and pineal. Please remember that we always strive for balance in our practice. This means that when you do this exercise, it is good to gently challenge yourself, but not to overdo it. It is always fine to shorten the duration of an exercise. You can also modify an exercise to your special needs by changing the range of motion.

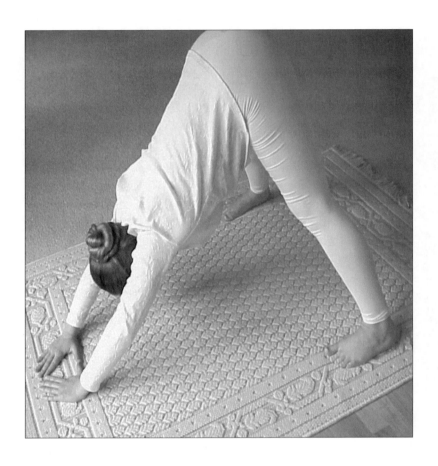

Dog Stretch for Total Body

Time
One to five minutes.

Physical Position
This is a standing position.

Instruction
Bring the feet about shoulder width apart with the feet creating a right angle to the plane of the body. Bend from the waist and place the hands on the floor. Hands are narrower than shoulder width apart. Have the thumb tips touching if possible. Elbows and knees are straight and the head is in line with the upper arms. Tilt the pelvis forward and push down through the shoulders, keeping equal weight on the hands and feet. Hold the position. Long Slow Deep Breathing.

Comments
It energizes the sciatic nerve and the power center at the navel point. It is a good total body stretch. It builds nervous system strength. Please remember that we always strive for balance in our practice. This means that when you do this exercise, it is good to gently challenge yourself, but not to overdo it. It is always fine to shorten the duration of an exercise. You can also modify an exercise to your special needs by changing the range of motion.

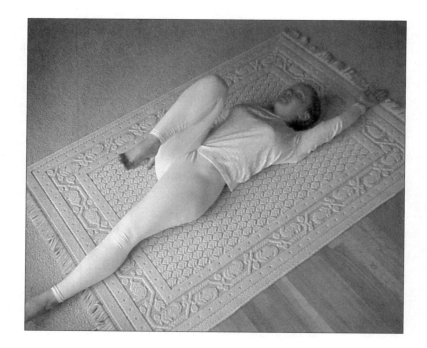

Cross Crawl Exercise for Brain Balance

Time

One to five minutes.

Physical Position

Lie flat on your back with the arms by the sides and the palms down.

Instruction

This is a moving exercise. Inhale as you bring the right knee up to the chest and at the same time bring the left arm back overhead on the ground in a backstroke motion. Exhale and return the arm and leg to the ground flat. Switch legs and arms. Use the opposite arm and opposite leg. Alternate with deep, powerful breathing.

Comments

This exercise energizes your power center at the navel point. It is a good body stretch that helps you to overcome boredom and fatigue. It is good for brain balance and helps to regulate elimination. Please remember that we always strive for balance in our practice. This means that when you do this exercise, it is good to gently challenge yourself, but not to overdo it. It is always fine to shorten the duration of an exercise. You can also modify an exercise to your special needs by changing the range of motion.

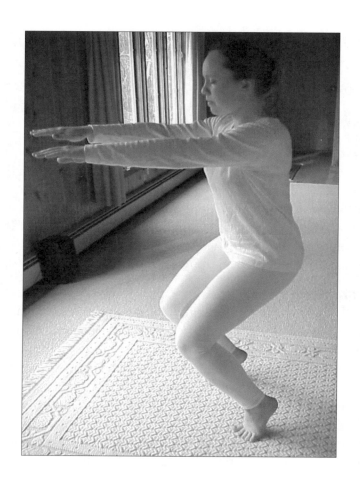

Standing Toe Raises for Knee Strength

Time

One to three minutes.

Physical Position

This is a standing position. Have the feet shoulder width apart with the feet at a right angle to the body.

Instruction

Bring the arms up parallel to the ground with the palms flat and shoulder width apart. Rise up on tiptoes. This is the inhale position. Exhale and staying on the toes, push the seat out and keep the chest lifted, bend the knees until the thighs are about parallel to the floor. Inhale up and exhale down, stay high on the toes as best you can.

Comments

This is good for overall circulation. It strengthens the thighs and is wonderful for strengthening weak knees. Please remember that we always strive for balance in our practice. This means that when you do this exercise, it is good to gently challenge yourself, but not to overdo it. It is always fine to shorten the duration of an exercise. You can also modify an exercise to your special needs by changing the range of motion.

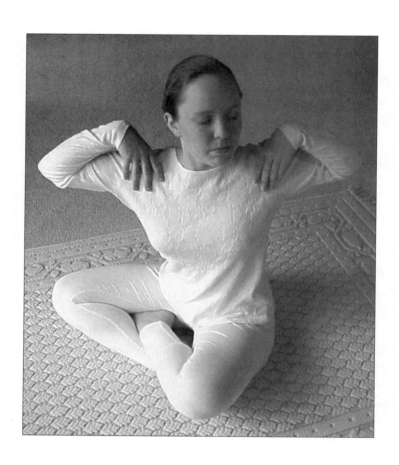

Washing Machine for the Waist

Time
One to three minutes.

Physical Position
Sit comfortably cross-legged. Bring the hands on the shoulders, fingers in front and thumbs in back.

Instruction
Inhale and twist the torso left and then exhale and twist the torso right. Keep the chest up high with the chin level to the ground. Let the head travel with the shoulders.

Comments
This exercise loosens and tones the waist and torso. It opens the nerve channels on either side of the spine. Please remember that we always strive for balance in our practice. This means that when you do this exercise, it is good to gently challenge yourself, but not to overdo it. It is always fine to shorten the duration of an exercise. You can also modify an exercise to your special needs by changing the range of motion.

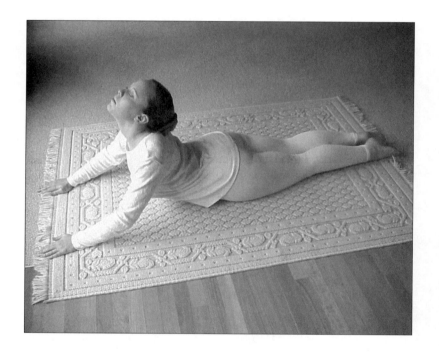

Cobra Stretch for Spine & Heart

Time

One to three minutes.

Physical Position

Lie down flat on the stomach. Bring the chin on the ground with the palms down on your mat underneath and slightly forward of the shoulders. Have the legs as close together as possible with the tops of the feet on the ground.

Instruction

This is a stationary position. Inhale and raise the head up, chest up and now smoothly push yourself up. Make sure the arms are shoulder width apart, elbows a little bent, fingers pointing forward, shoulders rolled back and down, chest high and head back. The whole pelvic area is on the ground. You can be resting on the forearms if it is more comfortable for you. Long Slow Deep Breathing.

Comments

It opens the diaphragm and chest. It energizes your power center at the navel. It opens your compassion center at the heart. It is a great stretch for the total spine. It adjusts the internal organs. It benefits the kidneys and adrenal glands. Please remember that we always strive for balance in our practice. This means that when you do this exercise, it is good to gently challenge yourself, but not to overdo it. It is always fine to shorten the duration of an exercise. You can also modify an exercise to your special needs by changing the range of motion.

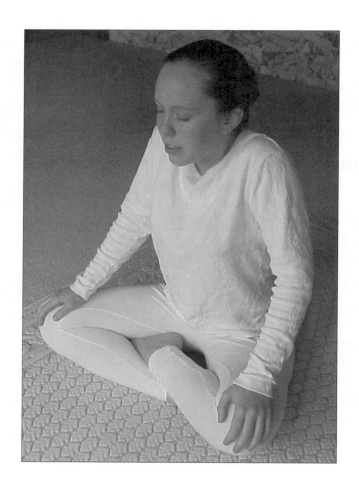

Shoulder Rolls for Upper Back & Shoulders

Time

One to three minutes.

Physical Position

Sit comfortably cross-legged. Bring the hands on the knees.

Instruction

Roll the shoulders together in big, slow, smooth circles. Inhale as you roll forward and up. Exhale as you roll back and down.

Comments

This exercise loosens tight shoulders and upper back. It opens the chest and your compassion center at the heart. Please remember that we always strive for balance in our practice. This means that when you do this exercise, it is good to gently challenge yourself, but not to overdo it. It is always fine to shorten the duration of an exercise. You can also modify an exercise to your special needs by changing the range of motion.

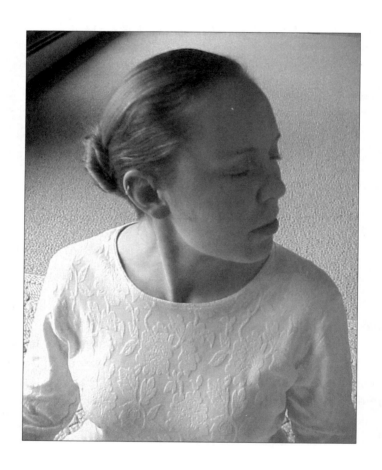

Neck Turns for Throat and Neck

Time

One to three minutes.

Physical Position

Sit comfortably cross-legged. Have the hands in the lap or at the knees.

Instruction

Inhale and slowly turn the head to the left. Exhale and slowly turn the head to the right. Keep the chin level to the ground and coordinate the breath with the motion. Long Slow Deep Breathing.

Comments

This exercise relaxes the neck and shoulders and back of the head. It helps the thyroid, parathyroid, pituitary and pineal glands. It opens your communication center at the throat.

Please remember that we always strive for balance in our practice. This means that when you do this exercise, it is good to gently challenge yourself, but not to overdo it. It is always fine to shorten the duration of an exercise. You can also modify an exercise to your special needs by changing the range of motion.

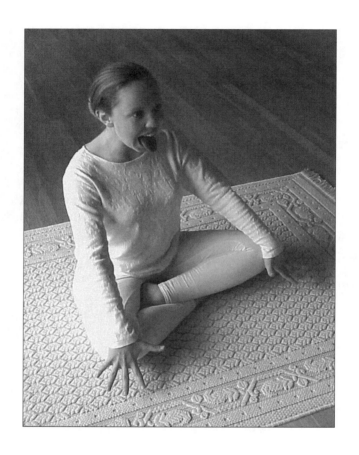

Lion Face for Fun

Time

Briefly held.

Physical Position

Sit comfortably cross-legged. Bring the hands on the knees.

Instruction

Open the mouth and stick the tongue out. Eyes are wide and wild, hand are in claws.

Comments

This fun position relaxes the face, relaxes the throat and makes you smile! Please remember that we always strive for balance in our practice. This means that when you do this exercise, it is good to gently challenge yourself, but not to overdo it. It is always fine to shorten the duration of an exercise. You can also modify an exercise to your special needs by changing the range of motion.

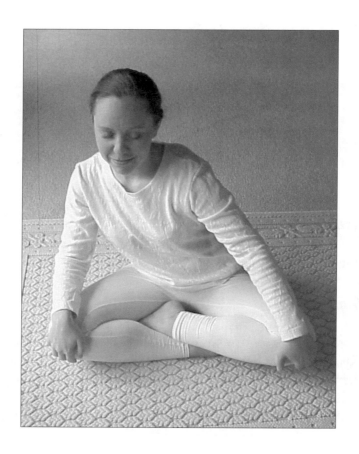

Exercise for Lower Back & Elimination

Time

One to three minutes in each direction

Physical Position

Sit comfortably cross-legged. Grasp the knees with the hands.

Instruction

This is a moving position. Tilt the pelvis back, then lean to the left, then arch and lean forward, then lean to the right. Keep the chin level in all positions. Continue the grinding for half the amount of time in one direction, then reverse and go the other direction. Normal Breath.

Comments

This exercise is great for lower back and hips. It helps make elimination regular. Please remember that we always strive for balance in our practice. This means that when you do this exercise, it is good to gently challenge yourself, but not to overdo it. It is always fine to shorten the duration of an exercise. You can also modify an exercise to your special needs by changing the range of motion.

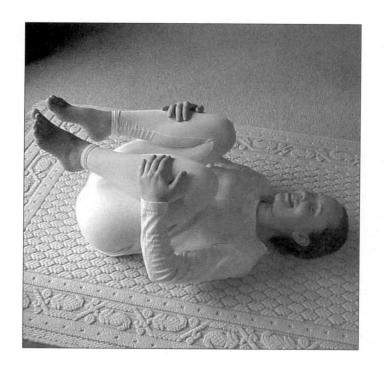

Exercise for Lower Back & Energy Recovery

Time

One to five minutes.

Physical Position

Lie flat on your back and draw both your knees up to your chest. Keep the head flat on the ground and wrap your hands around your shins or the thighs underneath the bent knees.

Instruction

Lie flat on your back and draw both your knees up to your chest. Keep the head flat on the ground and wrap your hands around your shins or in your thighs underneath the bent knees. Very gently draw the knees to the chest in a slow and easy (not jerking) pull and release rhythm. As you do the exercise, consciously relax the lower back. Normal Breath.

Comments

This exercise relieves tension in the lower back, especially after a long day on your feet. It releases stored energy for healing the body. Please remember that we always strive for balance in our practice. This means that when you do this exercise, it is good to gently challenge yourself, but not to overdo it. It is always fine to shorten the duration of an exercise. You can also modify an exercise to your special needs by changing the range of motion.

Chapter 2

 # *Basic Breaths*

Breath Overview

Yoga breathing exercises are among my favorite techniques to teach, simply because they are so effective and so accessible. You do not need any special place, or equipment to bring the breath into your conscious control. By bringing the breath into your conscious control, you can lead yourself into any number of beneficial states of being. You can do yoga breaths that can result in a calm and quiet body and mind, an energized and stimulated nervous system, an engaged intuitive capability and many other results as well.

The Yogi's view on the breath is quite interesting. You are a finite being - you have a certain life span, a certain amount of hours in the day, a certain amount of energy and activity that you can accomplish within a certain period of time. The view of the yogis' is that you have an infinite amount of energy, called prana, which is available to you. This energy, very much like chi in the Traditional Chinese Medicine model, is invisible, indivisible, and limitless. You can draw on that energy with the breath. It is the actual motion of the breath along with the cadence, rhythm, stroke and ratio of inhale and exhale that brings in the "prana" and qualifies how the body and mind will use that energy.

Normally you breathe about fifteen times per minute. Routinely, we will consciously slow the breath down to six breaths per minute and, with practice, down to one breath per minute. As part of the theory of breath, the Yogi's say that your life is measured in the number of breaths that you have to take in life. So, technically, you can extend life by slowing the breath down on a regular basis. In any event, with the stress reducing qualities of controlled breath, you will improve your health and well being, as well as the overall quality of life by practicing yoga breathing.

My personal experience is that your lung capacity will increase by practicing yoga and yoga breathing exercises. This leads to a generally more relaxed way of life when you are not practicing yoga. You will naturally breathe more slowly even when you have not brought your breath into your conscious control.

You can even be in a hurry and stay relatively more relaxed if you can slow the breath down in stressful situations! Practice of the yoga breaths in this book will definitely help bring greater control of the emotional and energy states in your life.

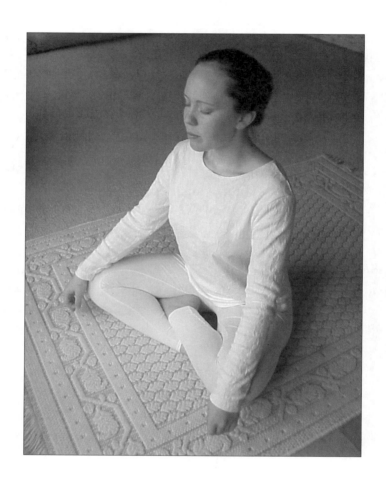

Long Slow Deep Breathing

Affirmation or Sounds

Any simple word repetition like "I am" or "Love Is" will help you keep your mental focus on the breath as you practice. Inhale "I" exhale "Am".

Time

Three to eleven minutes.

Physical position

Sit comfortably cross-legged on the floor or sit upright in chair with both feet flat on the ground. Hands can be folded in the lap or in the gyan mudra hand position (index finger and thumb touching) with the arms straight and the edges of the hands at the knees. This breath is used with different postures as well.

Instruction

This is the foundation of all breathing techniques. All inhales and exhales are done through the nose in a 1:1 ratio (inhale and exhale are equal in length). Six breaths a minute or slower will create a relaxation response in the body, help you to access your intuitive, problem solving capacity, adjust the spine and facilitate elimination. The breath is done by inhaling, and relaxing the diaphragm down and out; continue inhaling into the upper chest. Exhale, upper chest falls, diaphragm comes up and in at last. Keep the breath smooth in transition, not holding the breath in or out.

With the eyes gently closed and focused at the root of the nose, inhale through the nose and exhale through the nose, begin long, slow, deep breathing. Make the breath very smooth in transition, in other words do not hold the breath in or out. When the lungs are full, empty them and when the lungs are empty, fill them again. Your breath target rate is 4 to 6 complete breaths a minute. If you can slow the breath down even more with comfort then that is wonderful.

At the end

Inhale deeply, briefly hold the breath, and then relax.

Comments

This invaluable technique is the basic building block of all yoga breaths. It will calm you and sensitize your own self to your thoughts, your surroundings, and the natural flow of energies within and outside of the self. Yogi Bhajan has commented that this technique, as taught on the "Breathe Alaska" video that I have produced, is excellent for helping with digestive and blood disorders. The video is a useful tool for learning and practicing this breathing technique.

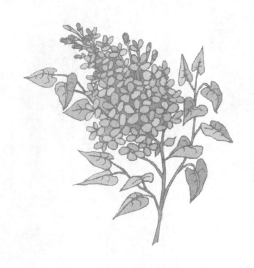

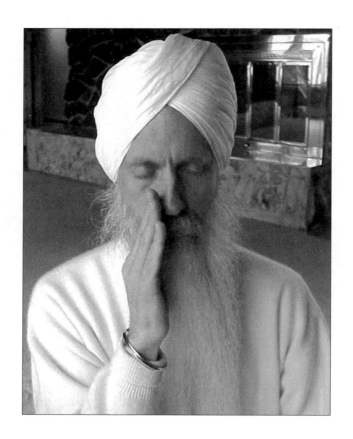

Calming Breath

Affirmation or Sounds

Any simple word repetition like "I am" or "Love Is" will help you keep your mental focus on the breath as you practice. Inhale "I" exhale "Am".

Time

Three to eleven minutes.

Physical position

Sit comfortably cross-legged on the floor or sit upright in chair with both feet flat on the ground. Hands can be folded in the lap or in the gyan mudra hand position (index finger and thumb touching) with the arms straight and the edges of the hands at the knees.

Instruction

This is left nostril only breathing. All inhales and exhales are done through the nose in a 1:1 ratio (inhale and exhale are equal in length). Six breaths a minute or slower will create a relaxation response in the body, help you to access your intuitive, problem solving capacity, adjust the spine and facilitate elimination. The breath is long slow and deep and is done by inhaling, and relaxing the diaphragm down and out; continue inhaling into the upper chest. Exhale, upper chest falls, diaphragm comes up and in at last. Keep the breath smooth in transition, not holding the breath in or out.

With the eyes gently closed and focused at the root of the nose, close off the right nostril and inhale through the left nostril and exhale through the left nostril. Make the breath very smooth in transition, in other words do not hold the breath in or out. When the lungs are full, empty them and when the lungs are empty, fill them again. Your breath target rate is 4 to 6 complete breaths a minute. If you can slow the breath down even more with comfort, then that is wonderful.

At the end

Inhale deeply, briefly hold the breath, and then relax.

Comments

This is long and deep "moon side" breathing for when you are upset, agitated or angry. It will cool you, calm you and slow you down. If the breath is done for a long enough time, it will allow you to be in the right brain hemisphere.

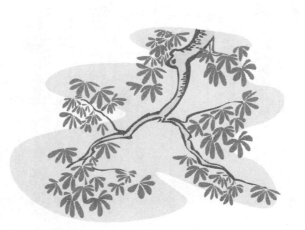

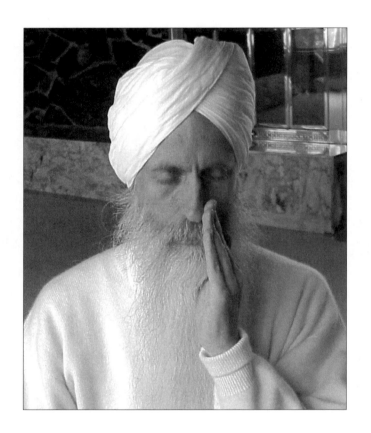

Energizing Breath

Affirmation or Sounds

Any simple word repetition like "I am" of "Love Is" will help you keep your mental focus on the breath as you practice. Inhale "I" exhale "Am".

Time

Three to eleven minutes.

Physical position

Sit comfortably cross-legged on the floor or sit upright in chair with both feet flat on the ground. Hands can be folded in the lap or in the gyan mudra hand position (index finger and thumb touching) with the arms straight and the edges of the hands at the knees.

Instruction

This is right nostril only breathing. All inhales and exhales are done through the nose in a 1:1 ratio (inhale and exhale are equal in length). Six breaths a minute or slower will create a relaxation response in the body, help you to access your intuitive, problem solving capacity, adjust the spine and facilitate elimination. The breath is long slow and deep and is done by inhaling, and relaxing the diaphragm down and out; continue inhaling into the upper chest. Exhale, upper chest falls, diaphragm comes up and in at last. Keep the breath smooth in transition, not holding the breath in or out.

With the eyes gently closed and focused at the root of the nose, close off the left nostril and inhale through the right nostril and exhale through the right nostril. Make the breath very smooth in transition, in other words do not hold the breath in or out. When the lungs are full, empty them and when the lungs are empty, fill them again. Your breath target rate is 4 to 6 complete breaths a minute. If you can slow the breath down even more with comfort, then that is wonderful.

At the end

Inhale deeply, briefly hold the breath, and then relax.

Comments

This is long and deep "sun" side breathing, for when you are cold, tired, unenthusiastic. It will warm the body, energize you and, if done for a long enough time, will allow you to be in the left brain hemisphere.

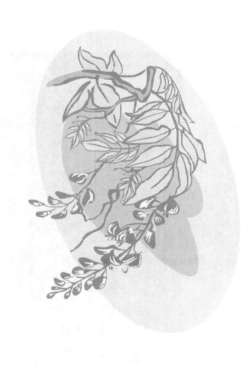

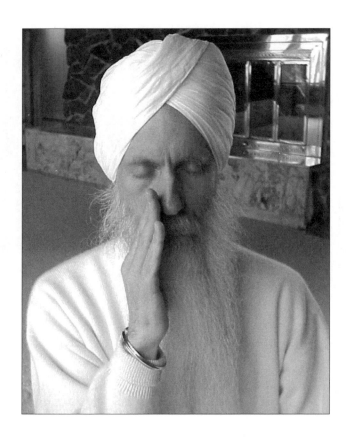

Balanced Breath

Affirmation or Sounds

Any simple affirmation like "I Am" or "Love Is" will help you keep your mental focus on the breath as you practice.

Time

Three to eleven minutes.

Physical position

Sit comfortably cross-legged on the floor or sit upright in chair with both feet flat on the ground. One hand will rest in the lap as the other hand closes alternate nostrils.

Instruction

This alternate nostril breathing technique is long slow deep breathing. You breathe long slow and deep as you switch breathing through opposite nostrils. All inhales and exhales are done through the nose in a 1:1 ratio (inhale and exhale are equal in length). Just like regular long slow deep breathing, this technique, at six breaths a minute or slower, will create a relaxation response in the body, help you to access your intuitive, problem solving capacity, adjust the spine and facilitate elimination. As in long slow deep breathing, you will inhale, relaxing the diaphragm down and out; continue inhaling into the upper chestexhale, upper chest falls, diaphragm comes up and in at last. Keep the breath smooth in transition, not holding the breath in or out.

Have the eyes gently closed and focused at the root of the nose, close off the right nostril as pictured and inhale through the left nostril and then close of the left nostril and exhale through the right nostril. Now reverse the pattern, close off the left nostril and inhale through the right nostril and then close of the right nostril and exhale through the left nostril. Inhale left (closing the right), exhale right (closing the left), inhale right (closing the left), exhale left (closing the right)…

Make the breath very smooth in transition, in other words do not hold the breath in or out. When the lungs are full, empty them and when the lungs are empty, fill them again. Your breath target rate is 4 to 6 complete breaths a minute. If you can slow the breath down even more with comfort, then that is wonderful. If you find that one nostril is a little blocked then allow a small bit of air in through the opposite nostril so you can keep the all the inhales and exhales equal in length.

At the end

Inhale deeply, briefly hold the breath, and then relax.

Comments

It will revitalize the nervous system. It helps to balance the brain hemispheres and can provide a nice transition between mental tasks and can clear off the effects of a busy day. This is a good breath to do before concentrating on a mental task or before meditation.

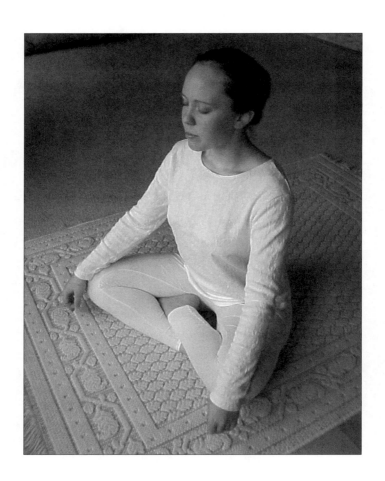

Cooling Breath

Affirmation or Sounds

Any simple word repetition like "I am" or "Love Is" will help you keep your mental focus on the breath as you practice. Inhale "I" exhale "Am".

Time

Three to eleven minutes.

Physical position

Sit comfortably cross-legged on the floor or sit upright in chair with both feet flat on the ground. Hands can be folded in the lap or in the gyan mudra hand position (index finger and thumb touching) with the arms straight and the edges of the hands at the knees.

Instruction

This breathing technique is long slow deep breathing inhaling through the mouth and exhaling through the nose. All inhales and exhales are done in a 1:1 ratio (inhale and exhale are equal in length). Just like regular long slow deep breathing, this technique at six breaths a minute or slower will cool you, soothe you and create a relaxation response in the body, help you to access your intuitive, problem solving capacity, adjust the spine and facilitate elimination. As in long slow deep breathing, you will inhale, relaxing the diaphragm down and out; continue inhaling into the upper chest. Exhale, upper chest falls, diaphragm comes up and in at last. Keep the breath smooth in transition, not holding the breath in or out.

Have the eyes gently closed and focused at the root of the nose, make a tunnel out of the tongue and inhale through this 'taco' tongue (if you are unable to roll the tongue simply point the tongue). Exhale through the nose. Make the breath very smooth in transition, in other words do not hold the breath in or out. When the lungs are full, empty them and when the lungs are empty, fill them again. Your breath target rate is 4 to 6 complete breaths a minute. If you can slow the breath down even more with comfort, then that is wonderful.

At the end

Inhale deeply, briefly hold the breath, and then relax.

Comments

This long slow deep breath (inhaling through the mouth in a tunnel tongue and exhaling through the nose) is the ultimate relaxing "chill out" breath. Good for "hot" conditions, irritability, impatience, or inappropriate anger.

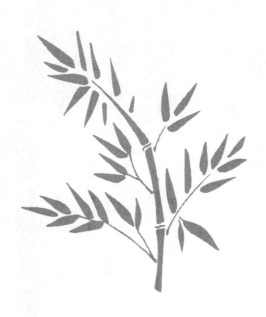

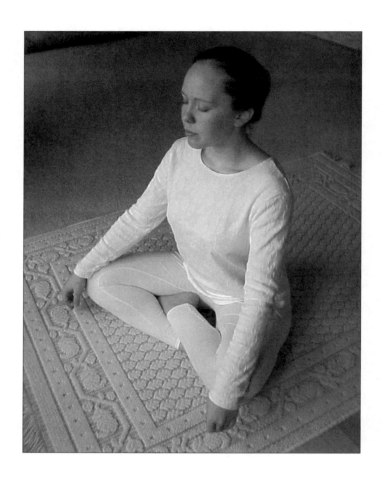

Ratio Breath for Go

Affirmation or Sounds

This is a counting breath in a 2:1 ratio. Count to eight on the inhale and count to four on the exhale. You can also use an affirmation like "I am, I am. I am, I am" on the inhale and "I am, I am" on the exhale. The sounds of "Sa Ta Na Ma" is also very useful for ratio counts of four. Example: Inhale "Sa Ta Na Ma" twice and exhale "Sa Ta Na Ma" once.

Time

Three to eleven minutes.

Physical position

Sit comfortably cross-legged on the floor or sit upright in chair with both feet flat on the ground. Hands can be folded in the lap or in the gyan mudra hand position (index finger and thumb touching) with the arms straight and the edges of the hands at the knees.

Instruction

This is an unequal breathing rhythm. All inhales and exhales are done through the nose in a 2:1 ratio (inhale is twice as long as the exhale). The breath is long slow and deep and is done by inhaling, and relaxing the diaphragm down and out; continue inhaling into the upper chest. Exhale, upper chest falls, diaphragm comes up and in at last. Keep the breath smooth in transition, not holding the breath in or out.

With the eyes gently closed and focused at the root of the nose, inhale slowly for a mental count of eight, and then exhale for a mental count of four. Make the breath very smooth in transition, in other words do not hold the breath in or out. When the lungs are full, empty them and when the lungs are empty, fill them again. If you can extend the count even more with comfort, then that is wonderful. For instance, you would inhale to a count of sixteen and exhale to a count of eight.

At the end

Inhale deeply, briefly hold the breath, and then relax.

Comments

This ratio breath will stimulate the sympathetic nervous system and really jazz you up.

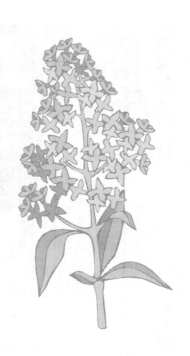

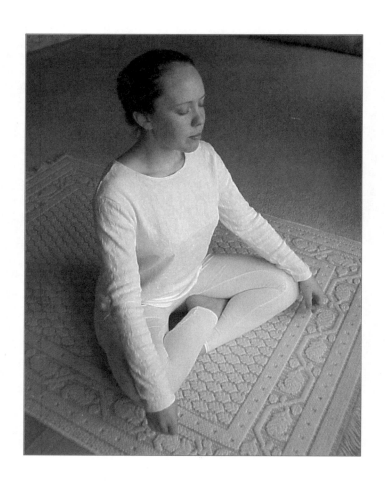

Ratio Breath for Slow

Affirmation or Sounds

This is a counting breath in a 1:2 ratio. Count to four on the inhale and count to eight on the exhale. You can also use an affirmation like "I am, I am" on the inhale and "I am, I am. I am, I am" on the exhale. The sounds of "Sa Ta Na Ma" is also very useful for ratio counts of four. Example: Inhale "Sa Ta Na Ma" once and exhale "Sa Ta Na Ma" twice.

Time

Three to eleven minutes.

Physical position

Sit comfortably cross-legged on the floor or sit upright in chair with both feet flat on the ground. Hands can be folded in the lap or in the gyan mudra hand position (index finger and thumb touching) with the arms straight and the edges of the hands at the knees.

Instruction

This is an unequal breathing rhythm. All inhales and exhales are done through the nose in a 1:2 ratio (inhale is half as long as the exhale). The breath is long slow and deep and is done by inhaling, and relaxing the diaphragm down and out; continue inhaling into the upper chest. Exhale, upper chest falls, diaphragm comes up and in at last. Keep the breath smooth in transition, not holding the breath in or out.

With the eyes gently closed and focused at the root of the nose, inhale slowly for a mental count of four and then exhale for a mental count of eight. Make the breath very smooth in transition, in other words do not hold the breath in or out. When the lungs are full, empty them and when the lungs are empty, fill them again. If you can extend the count even more with comfort, then that is wonderful. For instance, you would inhale to a count of eight and exhale to a count of sixteen.

At the end

Inhale deeply, briefly hold the breath, and then relax.

Comments

This ratio breath will stimulate the parasympathetic nervous system, slow you down and mellow you out.

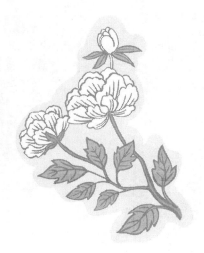

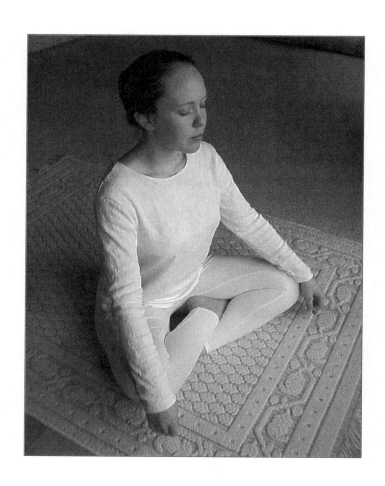

Segmented Breath for Depression

Affirmation or Sounds

This is a counting breath in a 4:1 ratio. Count to four on the segmented inhale and count to one, in one long exhale. You can also use an affirmation like "I am, I am" on the inhale and a single word like "Blissful" on the exhale.

Time

Three to eleven minutes.

Physical position

Sit comfortably cross-legged on the floor or sit upright in chair with both feet flat on the ground. Hands can be folded in the lap or in the gyan mudra hand position (index finger and thumb touching) with the arms straight and the edges of the hands at the knees.

Instruction

This is an unequal breathing rhythm done in segments or sniffs. All inhales and exhales are done through the nose in a 4:1 ratio (inhale is four times as long as the exhale). The breath is segmented into small equal sniff and is done by a small inhale, inhale, inhale, inhale and then a single long exhale. Keep the breath smooth in transition, not holding the breath in or out.

With the eyes gently closed and focused at the root

of the nose, inhale in four slow even and rhythmic segments. Exhale in one long slow even yet forceful breath. Make the breath very smooth in transition, in other words do not hold the breath in or out and be sure that the inhale is four times as long as the exhale. Use your complete lung capacity, when the lungs are full, empty them and when the lungs are empty, fill them again.

At the end

Inhale deeply, briefly hold the breath, and then relax.

Comments

This ratio breath can help alleviate minor depression.

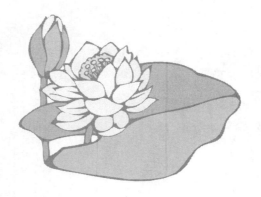

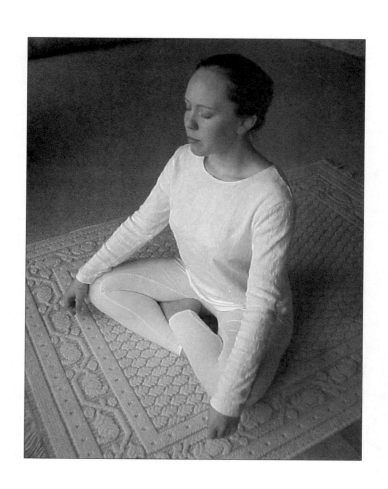

Segmented Breath for Anxiety

Affirmation or Sounds

This is a counting breath in a 1:2 ratio. Count to four on the segmented inhale and count to eight on the segmented exhale. You can also use an affirmation like "I am, I am" on the inhales and "I am, I am. I am, I am" on the exhales. The sounds of " Sa Ta Na Ma" is also very useful for ratio counts of four. Example: Inhale "Sa Ta Na Ma" once and exhale "Sa Ta Na Ma" twice.

Time

Three to eleven minutes.

Physical position

Sit comfortably cross-legged on the floor or sit upright in chair with both feet flat on the ground. Hands can be folded in the lap or in the gyan mudra hand position (index finger and thumb touching) with the arms straight and the edges of the hands at the knees.

Instruction

This is an unequal breathing rhythm done in segments or sniffs. All inhales and exhales are done through the nose in a 1:2 ratio (inhale is half as long as the exhale). The breath is segmented into small equal sniffs and is done by a small inhale, inhale, inhale, inhale and then twice as many exhales done in the same fashion. Keep the breath smooth in transition, not holding the breath in or out.

With the eyes gently closed and focused at the root of the nose, inhale in four slow even and rhythmic segments. Exhale in eight slow, even and rhythmic segments. Make the breath very smooth in transition, in other words do not hold the breath in or out. When the lungs are full, empty them and when the lungs are empty, fill them again. If you can extend the count even more with comfort, then that is wonderful. For instance, you would inhale in eight segments and exhale in sixteen segments.

At the end

Inhale deeply, briefly hold the breath, and then relax.

Comments

This segmented breath in a 1:2 ratio will stimulate the parasympathetic nervous system, and can help relieve anxiety.

Chapter 3

Heal Your Back Now!
Exercise Series

Kundalini Yoga is excellent for the back. My experience has shown me that it is particularly effective for congenital curvatures of the spine. In Kundalini Yoga we spend a lot of time working with the flexibility of the spine. We move the whole back in many different ways that you don't normally do in adult life. We use static stretching, range of motion movements, and also move energy through the spine. In addition, we work on the energy fields and learn and practice meditation techniques that clear and clarify the mind and emotions. The net result is a healthy and pain free back as well as the means to keep it that way!

The real solution to the physical part of most back problems lies in working with three specific areas of the body. To maintain a healthy lower back you must stretch the hamstrings, build the strength of the navel center, which is your power center, through abdominal strengthening, and move the back in a variety of ways. This exercise series works in all these areas. This exercise series is on the video "Heal Your Back Now!" Start by intoning the mantra "Ong Namo Guru Dev Namo" three times for saluting your highest consciousness.

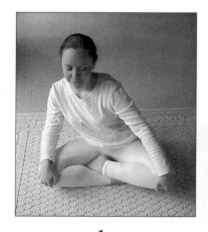

1

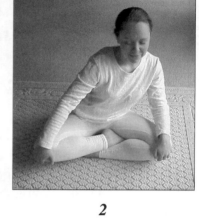

2

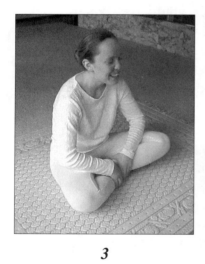

3

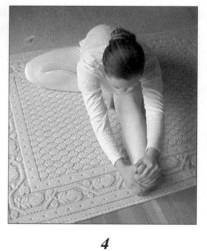

4

1 *Pelvic Grind Left*

Place your hands on your knees and begin grinding yourself in a big circle going to the left. Lift the chest up high as you come forward and let the chest collapse and the pelvis tilt backwards as you go back. Keep the chin level to the ground in both positions. Normal Breath. (ninety seconds)

2 *Pelvic Grind Right*

Continue grinding yourself in a big smooth circle going to the right. Lift the chest up high as you come forward and let the chest collapse and the pelvis tilt backwards as you go back. Keep the chin level to the ground in both positions. Normal Breath. (ninety seconds)

3 *Basic Spine Flex*

Place the hands on the shins right above the ankles. Grasp the shins firmly and now inhale through the nose and lift the chest up high and tilt the pelvis forward. Now exhale through the nose, collapse the chest and gently tilt the pelvis the opposite way. Inhale up and exhale back. Inhale up and exhale back. Inhale up and exhale back. Continue. Remember to lift the chest up high on each inhale and keep the chin level to the ground in both positions. (three minutes)

4 *Front Stretch Left*

Now stretch your left leg out in front of you straight; right foot against the inner thigh of the left leg. With both hands, stretch forward then down over the left leg. Hold on to your shin, ankle or foot with both hands. Keep the chin at a right angle to the chest. Stretch forward and then down, until you feel gently challenged by the stretch. Hold it steady; we like to do static stretching in Kundalini Yoga. Long Slow Deep Breathing. (ninety seconds)

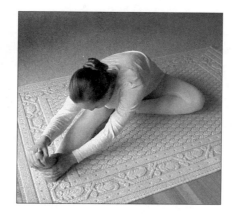

5

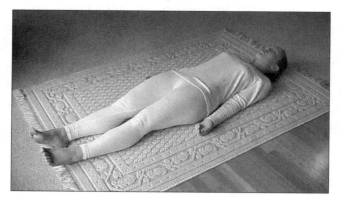

6

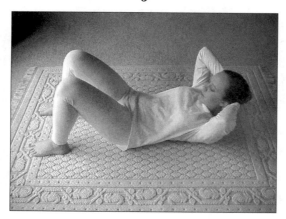

7

5 *Front Stretch Right*

Now stretch your right leg out in front of you straight, left foot against the inner thigh of the right leg. With both hands, stretch forward then down over the right leg. Hold on to your shin, ankle or foot with both hands. Keep the chin at a right angle to the chest. Stretch forward and then down, until you feel gently challenged by the stretch. Hold it steady, we like to do static stretching in Kundalini Yoga. Long Slow Deep Breathing. (ninety seconds)

6 *Short Rest*

Come out of position and rest on your back. Lie down flat, have the arms by the side palms up, with the eyes gently closed and the breath soft and normal. Have the knees up slightly for comfort, if needed. Normal Breath. (thirty seconds)

7 *Yoga Crunch*

Bring knees up and have your feet flat against the floor. Make the hands into a basket by interlacing them and placing them behind the head. We are going to doing a six-count movement both up and down. So now lift the head off the ground and remember to just support the head with the hands. Try not to pull on the neck with the hands or arms. And now, tilt the pelvis so that the lower back is flat against the floor. We want to keep the lower back flat through out the exercise. In this position, inhale slowly and now exhale and slowly curl up tightening the abdominal muscles... One... two...three...four...five...six. Now inhale and slowly loosen the abdominal as you go back.

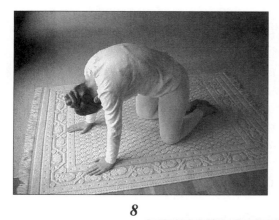

8

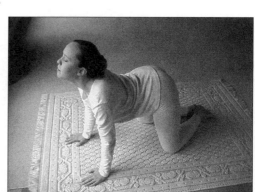

8

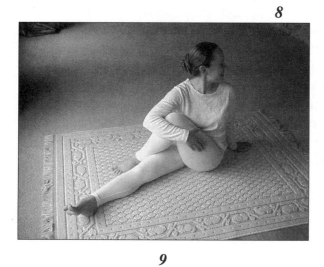

9

One...two...three...four...five...six. Good, keep the head up in both positions. This will help you keep the lower back flat against the floor. Continue, go slow and concentrate your breaths' energy right at your navel point. Imagine as though you are breathing in and out through the navel. This will help you concentrate on this area of the body. (two minutes)

8 *Cow-Cat*

Draw the knees up to the chest and rock yourself up. The hands are straight down from the shoulders with the fingers pointing forward and the elbows locked straight. If your wrists bother you, then make your hands into fists, and place the knuckles on the ground. The knees are straight down from the hips and are separated by about six inches. Toes are uncurled.

Your neck is going to stay in line with your upper spine in this exercise, so the face is almost parallel to the floor, just slightly tilted up. This is a two- part motion. You are going to inhale and tilt the pelvis forward in cow position. Now exhale, tilt the pelvis the opposite way and at the same time push up through the shoulders in cat position.

The head remains fairly stable. Inhale through the nose into cow, and exhale through the nose into cat. Continue. Make the motion very smooth in transition. When you have reached your full range of motion in one position then initiate the other position. (two minutes)

9 *Half-Spinal Twist Left*

Come out of position, sit down and stretch your legs out in front of you straight. Bring the left knee up. Cross the left foot over the right leg placing the foot flat on the floor. Take the left hand and bring it all the way back down and behind you on the left side. Take the right arm and wrap it around the left leg. Straighten up. Keeping the chin level to the ground, turn the chin all the way left. Chest up high, left shoulder and chin all the way left. Long Slow Deep Breathing. (one minute)

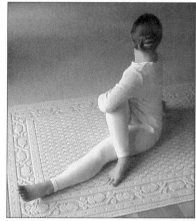

10

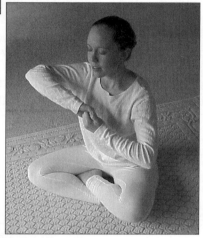

11

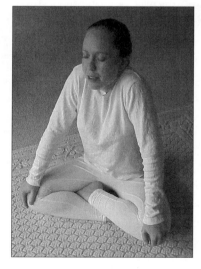

12

10 Half Spinal Twist Right

Straighten the legs. Bring the right knee up. Cross the right foot over the left leg placing the foot flat on the floor. Take the right hand and bring it all the way back down and behind you on the right side. Take the left arm and wrap it around the right leg. Straighten up. Keeping the chin level to the ground, turn the chin all the way right. Chest up high, right shoulder and chin all the way right .Long Slow Deep Breathing. (one minute)

11 Shoulder Teeter-Totters

Sit cross-legged, and hook the hands together like you have bear claws. The left can be either facing in or out. Keep the arms parallel to the ground to begin and use the heart center as a pivot for your teeter-totter, with hands four to six inches out from the chest. Inhale and lift the left elbow up and the right elbow goes down, exhale and the left elbow goes down and the right elbow goes up. Continue. Let all the motion happen in the shoulders and arms without leaning from side to side. (one minute) At the end, inhale the arms parallel to the ground. Pull on the grip, hold the breath. Exhale, relax the arms.

12 Shoulder Shrugs

Stretch your legs out for a moment and shake them out. Sit cross-legged again and bring your hands out to your knees. Grasp the knees with the hands and now inhale through the nose and lift the shoulders up high and now exhale and let the shoulders drop. Go at any pace that is comfortable to you, from a moderate to a rapid pace. Just let the whole shoulder girdle drop down. Inhale up and exhale down. Continue. (one minute)

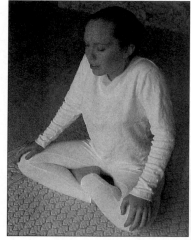

13

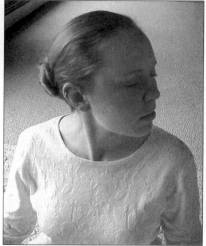

14

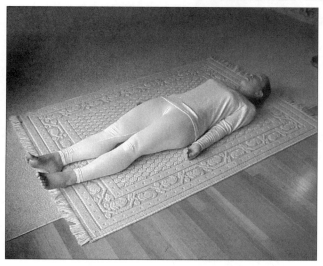

15

13 Shoulder Rolls

Now inhale and lift the shoulders up high, hold the breath. Exhale, and relax the shoulders down. Now begin rolling the shoulders in big circles. Normal Breath. (one minute)

14 Neck Rolls Or Turns.

We will roll the head and neck now. If you are not comfortable with rolling your head you can turn your head from side to side keeping the chin level to the ground. Now slowly begin rolling the head in a large smooth circle in one direction, breath is relaxed. Normal Breath. (thirty seconds) Consciously relax the neck, throat and shoulders as you roll. Now reverse direction. Normal Breath. (thirty seconds)

15 Deep Relaxation

Come out of position and rest on your back. Lie down flat, have the arms by the side palms up, with the eyes gently closed and the breath soft and normal. Have the knees up slightly for comfort, if needed.

Chapter 4

Meditation
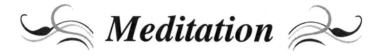

Why And How To Meditate

Why meditate? My teacher, Yogi Bhajan, said in order to live in Alaska you have to do one of two things. You either must meditate a lot or you must drink a lot of alcohol! The reason being that this is a highly energetic environment. Some of it has to do with the extreme night and day cycle, but it's primarily because of our closeness to magnetic north, and our closeness to the tallest mountain in North America. Denali is a very powerful presence. All this energy creates a lot of internal pressure that needs to be released. Of course, this is not only true for Alaska. The pressures and stresses of our fast paced Western lifestyle make meditation a virtual necessity no matter where you live.

There are many reasons to meditate. Meditation can help you handle stress, build intuition and increase self-awareness. My personal view is that meditation is as essential as daily bathing and serves a very similar function. Generally you do not have to take a bath or shower on a daily basis because your body is dirty. You may have some extra salts on your body that are creating an undesirable odor but unless you are a hard playing seven year old, then you actually bathe or shower for another reason. This reason is that bathing makes you feel good! You feel refreshed, renewed and rejuvenated. The reason for this has to do with the blood circulation in your capillaries and the capacity of water to hold, carry and remove tired and stagnant energy.

Meditation has a very similar function. It provides a way for you to process your mental thoughts and energetic pre-dispositions. The result is that, just like bathing, you feel relaxed and refreshed, renewed and rejuvenated. The long-term benefits of meditation are even more profound. Potentially, you can make your life much smoother and bring your life into alignment with your soul's purpose.

Meditation works in two ways; you have the opportunity to watch your mind and involve yourself in a mental process of self-correction. No matter what kind of meditation that you are doing, you are sitting with yourself and you can become an observer of your thoughts. It can be silent/observational meditation, breath centered, sound/mantra or mudra (hand position) related meditation. Your mind will be working and you will be involved not only in what you are doing but what is happening as you are doing it. In other words, you have the opportunity to watch and observe your mind as you think. It becomes a very interesting act in conscious self-awareness. It can provide you with a lot of invaluable insights about yourself. Most of the time, we are so busy doing; we do not take the time to record how it all feels and how the doings have affected us physically, mentally and emotionally.

Meditation also involves a process. It is a very popular misconception that you have to empty your mind to meditate and you have to concentrate perfectly. Even one of the greatest mystics and meditators of modern times, a man called Ramakrishna, would not empty his mind. This is a man who would see birds flying overhead in a flock and would fall into a deep state of meditation/trance. He would experience ecstasy, from the beauty of seeing the birds flying so freely and carefree. But he always said I never let myself go completely. I always keep a little bit of ego with me, some identification, so I can really appreciate what I'm experiencing. Otherwise I would be so merged, I wouldn't know it was me that was doing it! A person like Ramakrishna is very rare. Mostly we cannot escape our thoughts as normal human beings but we can involve our thoughts in a process. This process of meditation involves using a focal point.

A focal point is a reference that you can use as the mind wanders during meditation. A focal point can be a flow of energy, a breath rhythm, an eye or hand position, or sounds. It also can be a combination of any of these focuses. When the mind wanders, it can be very interesting to observe where the mind goes and then, when you realize that you have lost your focal point, to bring it gently back into focus. This is the process of meditation, which is extremely valuable.

It is valuable because it allows you on a conscious and unconscious level to correct a mental pattern that may be keeping you from a realizing your potential as a human being and living a smooth, happy life. Very simply, you have a tendency for being over projective or over protective. Either you are, by nature, a risk taker or you avoid risk. This tendency has come from your family background, your cultural and environmental background. In order to make good decisions, balance is needed. You need balance between your projective and protective self.

The very act of gently bringing the mind back to

focal point will help to balance your tendency. This is accomplished by getting into the habit of "zeroing" your mind. The focal point represents a "zero" or meditative/ neutral state. For instance, you'll think about your laundry, and then you'll think about your focal point. Then you'll burp and you'll think about lunch, you'll think about a discomfort in the body, and then you'll remember your focal point. Your mind will wander to your carpet and how it needs vacuuming, and then you'll think about changing your snow tires, and then you'll remember your focal point. The process is that every time you find yourself wandering off, you remind your mind of your center, of your resting-place. This focal point can be your neutral observation, or the breathing technique, or the sound/ mantra. It is this process that helps you with self-realization. This process works with your tendency to process things either more through your projective mind or more through your protective mind, so you can cultivate within you a habitual meditative mind. A meditative mind will make good balanced decisions and create a very smooth and happy life.

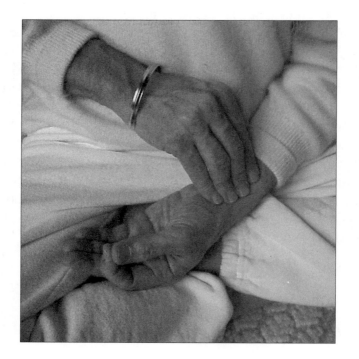

Meditation for Centering

Affirmation or Sounds

The sound of your heartbeat can be effectively linked with any two-word affirmation or mantra. Suggested words are "I am," or "Love is".

Time

Three to eleven minutes.

Physical Position

Sit comfortably cross-legged on the floor or sit upright in chair with both your feet flat on the ground. You will be using one of your hands for feeling your pulse at the wrist or the throat. The other hand stays relaxed at the knee or in the lap. Eyes are gently closed and focused at the brow point.

Instruction

Take the fingertips on one hand and place them on the upturned wrist of the other arm, with hands resting comfortably in your lap. If you cannot feel the pulse at the wrist, place the fingertips at the carotid artery at the throat. Simply feel and meditate on the pulse, linking up an internal affirmation or mantra with beat of your heart.
Breath is soft and relaxed.

At the end

Inhale deeply, briefly hold the breath, and then relax.

Comments

This meditation will bring you into very gentle focus. It is wonderful to do when you are feeling mentally scattered or emotionally drained. It will renew you with a sense of well being and soft, centered awareness.

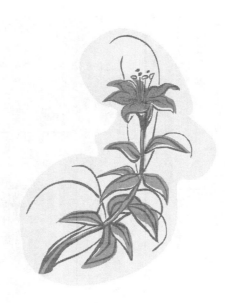

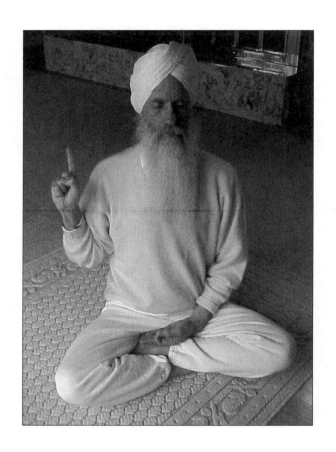

Meditation for Intuition

Affirmation or Sounds

This is a silent meditation with no affirmations or sounds.

Time

One to seven minutes.

Physical Position

Sit comfortably cross-legged on the floor or sit upright in chair with both your feet flat on the ground. Left hand is in the lap and the right arm is held out comfortably to the side. Eyes are gently closed and focused at the brow point.

Instruction

Make the right hand into a fist with the Jupiter finger (the index finger) extended and pointing straight up. The left hand is relaxed in the lap. Close your eyes and sit quietly, unmoving in this position. Let your breath slow down and self regulate.

At the end

Inhale deeply, hold the breath and stretch your right arm up as high as you can (keeping the fist and the pointed finger). After 15-20 seconds, powerfully exhale, inhale again, hold the breath and stretch every fiber of your body up. Again, after 15-20 seconds exhale powerfully and relax. Relax a couple of minutes and then shake your arms above your head for a few seconds to finish.

Comments

This meditation will help to develop your intuition. Intuition is when you know or sense something that you can't "logically" explain. It is one of the faculties of a person that has been awakened to their potential and has developed their awareness. Intuition combined with your rational thought process lets you know what to do within any given situation in a very effective and intelligent manner.

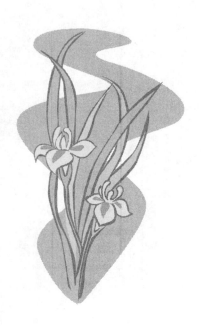

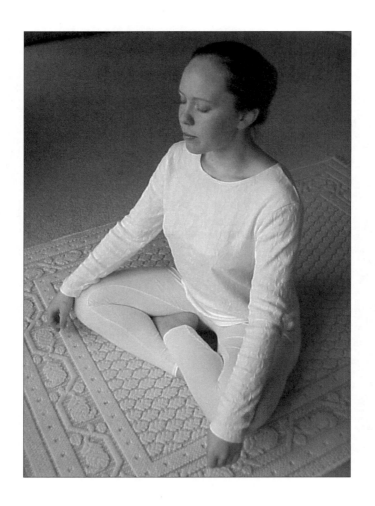

Meditation for Prosperity

Affirmation or Sounds

After the inhale, as you hold the breath in, you recite mentally "I am bountiful, I am blissful, I am beautiful." While you hold the breath out, you mentally recite, "Excel, excel, fearless."

Time

Three minutes.

Physical Position

Sit comfortably cross-legged on the floor or sit upright in chair with both feet flat on the ground. Hands can be folded in the lap or in the Gyan Mudra hand position (index finger and thumb touching) with the arms straight and the edges of the hands at the knees. Eyes are closed and pressed down looking as though you could see the center of the chin.

Instruction

Inhale deeply and hold the breath in and recite mentally "I am bountiful, I am blissful, I am beautiful." Exhale and while you hold the breath out, you mentally recite, "Excel, excel, fearless."

At the end

Inhale deeply, briefly hold the breath, and then relax.

Comments

This meditation can help to bring prosperity into your life. It can be practiced three to four times daily if desired. It is a wonderful desk meditation to refresh and recharge your self during the day.

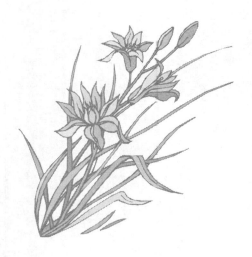

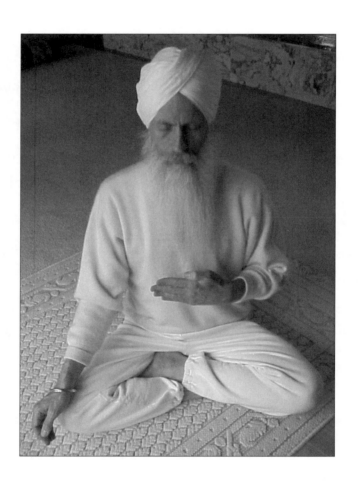

Meditation into Being

Affirmation or Sounds

I Am, I Am.

Time

Three to eleven minutes.

Physical Position

Sit comfortably cross-legged on the floor or sit up-right in chair with both your feet flat on the ground. You will be using your left hand for the movement while the right hand stays relaxed at the right knee or in the lap.

Instruction

Using the left hand, place it front of the heart cen-ter about six inches in front of the chest. As you say the mantra "I Am" out loud, bring the hand, with the palm facing your chest, in closer to the chest (about four inches away). On the second "I Am," move the hand away from the chest until it is about twelve inches out from the chest. Inhale through the nose and then bring the hand back to the beginning. position of being six inches in front of the chest. Continue this cycle.

At the end

Inhale deeply, briefly hold, then relax.

Comments

This meditation will bring you a relaxed and magnetic awareness of the your heart center and an identity that exists in the present moment. It takes care of the mental self-questioning of identity through a loop process of self-answering. You say "I Am" and if a subconscious question arises (I am what?) you answer to your own self "I Am." This self-education can be very healing.

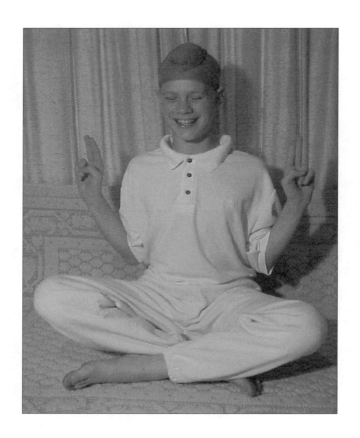

Smiling Buddha Meditation

Affirmation of Sounds

The sounds used in this meditation are "Sa Ta Na Ma." Translation is Life, Life ongoing, End of life, Renewal of life.

Time

Three to eleven minutes

Physical position

Sit comfortably cross-legged on the floor or sit upright in chair with both feet flat on the floor. Upper arms are held comfortably by the side with the elbows down and the hands facing forward with the thumb holding down both the ring and little fingers. Index and Tall finger are together and pointing up. Fingertips will be at about shoulder height or a little higher. Lift your chest up high. Keep the chin level to the ground and slightly tucked in. Eyes are closed and focused at the root of the nose. Most importantly, SMILE. Keep your smile for the entire meditation. It can be a Mona Lisa smile or a big goofy grin; it is your choice. Keep smiling!

Instruction

Concentrate the mantra "Sa Ta Na Ma" at the brow point (eyes focused at the root of the nose). Breath is normal.

At the end

Inhale deeply and stretch the arms overhead and the shake the hands vigorously.

Comments

This kriya brings lightness and peace. Use it when you are over stressed and over burdened.

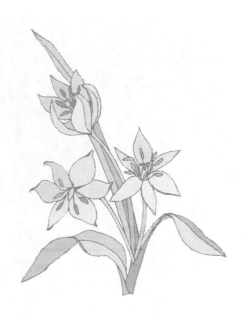

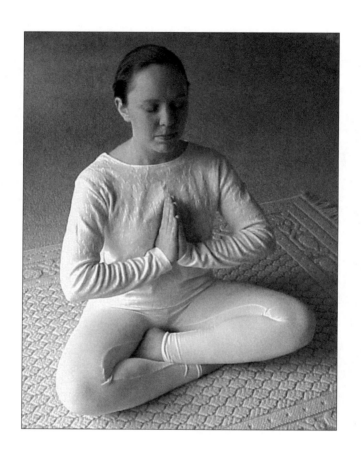

Meditation for Projected Healing

Affirmation or Sounds

This meditation uses a song as well as a mental concentration. The words to the song are "May the Long-time Sun shine upon you, all Love surround you and the pure Light within you, Guide your way on."

Time

Recite the words or sing the song as long as it takes to sing it through twice.

Physical Position

Sit comfortably cross-legged on the floor or sit up-right in chair with both your feet flat on the ground. Have the palms together with the base of the thumbs lightly pressed against the sternum. This will help you to concentrate.

Instruction

Sing the song as you mentally concentrate on a person. Sending healing energy to this person by visualizing them as being healthy and happy, as though they have already received and benefited from the energy and the kind thoughts that you are sending. If you are a feeling person, feel as though the person is sitting right in front of you and get the feeling that the person is happy and healthy. This works very well for conflict resolution as well. If you are having difficulty with a person at home or at work, you can really move the energy and open communication and perhaps even resolve the difficulty by singing them the song.

At the end

Inhale deeply, briefly hold the breath, and then relax.

Comments

This meditation will allow you to share energy, heal at a distance or resolve conflicts with other people.

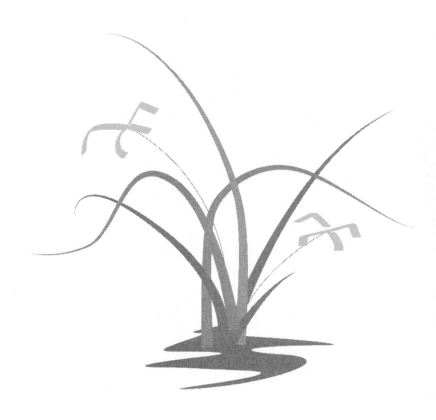

Chapter 5

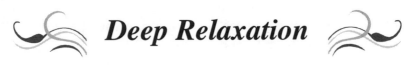 *Deep Relaxation*

The ability to deeply relax at bedtime or before a nap is a wonderful life enhancing skill to learn. As part of a class, deep relaxation is a real favorite among students and a very important part of a Kundalini Yoga class. The deep relaxation at the end of class typically runs for five to fifteen minutes. It gives the body, glandular system and nervous system an opportunity to re-balance. It is very relaxing and refreshing. It might be the best and most relaxed rest you get all day.

During the deep relaxation it is a good idea to really allow the body and mind relax. If you happen to fall asleep, it is OK. It is best to not actively scheme, plan and think. Here are three of the guided deep relaxation meditations that we use in class and that you can use at home before you nap or retire for the evening.

Part by part mental deep relaxation

Lie down flat on your back with arms by the side, palms up and the legs uncrossed. Breath is soft and normal. We will relax the body part by part mentally starting with the feet and working all the way up to the head. Follow my instructions and allow yourself to totally and completely relax. First relax the soles of the feet, tops of the feet, toes, heels and ankles. Now relax the legs, calves,

111

shins, knees and thighs. Relax the pelvic area, the hips, buttocks, abdomen and waist. Relax the hands, fingers, palms thumbs and wrists. Now relax the stomach, diaphragm, ribcage and chest. Relax the back, lower back; middle back, upper back and shoulders. Relax the throat and neck. Relax the face, the chin, lips, cheekbones, ears, temples, nose, eyes, forehead and scalp. Allow the body to totally and completely relax.

Part by Part Tension and Release Relaxation

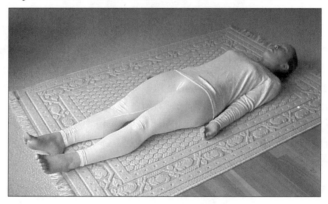

Lie down flat on your back with the arms by the sides, palms up and the legs uncrossed. Breath is soft and normal. We will use the tension and release method of relaxation. Follow my instructions and allow yourself to totally and completely relax.

First, press the toes away from the body and release. Now pull the toes back toward the head and release. Press the backs of the knees against your mat; tighten the thighs and release. Tighten the muscles in the buttocks, release. Tilt the pelvis, so the lower back is flat, release. Make tight fist out of the hands, release. Bring the fingertips up on the shoulders and make a biceps muscle, release, relax the arms down. Shrug the shoulders forward across the body, release. Pinch the shoulder blades together behind the back, release. Shrug the shoulders up to the ears, release and settle the shoulders in. Keeping the head on the ground, bring the chin down toward the collarbone, release. Keeping the head on the ground, lift the chin up and back, release. Keeping the head on the ground, turn the head from side to side until you find a comfortable place for your head. Now find that place. Scrunch up and tighten the face, mouth, nose, eyes and forehead, release. Take a deep inhale and with this exhale, let all the tension go in the body. Allow yourself to totally and completely relax.

Overall Relaxation with Guided Visualization

Lie down flat on your back with the arms by the side, palms up and the legs uncrossed. Breath is soft and normal. Now relax the body all at once. Let everything go all at one time. Allow your self to sink into your mat feeling heavy and relaxed throughout your entire body. Now bring yourself mentally to your favorite place of rest. It can be from your past or present. It can be in your own cozy bed at home or under a favorite tree, lying on a favorite beach or floating on a raft in a calm lake. Pick a place where you feel the most at peace with yourself, cozy, protected and secure. Now recreate this scene with as much detail as you can, all the smells, sounds and sights. Most of all recreate the feeling you have by being there. Now allow yourself to totally and completely relax.

Coming out of the Deep Relaxation

This routine will really help you adjust the body when coming out of a deep relaxation. It adjusts your spine, navel center point and nervous system so that you will feel more alert and together when you get up from your rest.

1. Roll your hands and a roll your feet.
2. Stretch the arms overhead, point the toes as well, and stretch.
3. Keeping the arms over head, bend your left leg by bringing the knee close to the chest and bring the knee over the straight right leg and twist the torso. Switch sides and bend your right leg by bringing your left knee close to the chest and then bring the knee over the straight left leg and twist the torso.
4. Rub the hands together and rub the soles of the feet together vigorously.
5. Draw the knees up to the chest and rock yourself up.

Foot Massage

Foot massage or Reflexology is an old a science as Kundalini Yoga. I learned foot massage from Yogi Bhajan and it is part of the tradition of Kundalini Yoga. The basis of foot massage is that you have seventy two thousand nerve endings on the bottom of your foot and they reflex to very specific parts of the body.

There are three benefits to foot massage. The first benefit is that foot massage is very relaxing. It soothes and helps to balance the nervous system. It is wonderful for tired, stressed and sick people.

The second benefit is that foot massage is lay diagnostic. When sore spots or "crystals" are found on the foot, it means that there is some energy blockage that relates to the reflex point on the foot. This can be a genetic condition or an acquired condition. In any event, it is probably something you know about yourself already and is not to be construed as a serious medical diagnosis. I have been teaching foot massage for three decades and I have only run across one person that has not had any crystals on the bottom of their feet. Crystals are mineral deposits on the nerve endings.

The third benefit of foot massage is that it is a legitimate healing modality. Healing touch acts as a catalyst for the body to heal itself. I have heard several

stories of disease remissions and alleviation of nagging physical problems using foot massage.

Foot massages can be light, heavy/therapeutic and

somewhere in the middle. We will aspire to the middle way. When you are massaging your partners' feet, mix your techniques of general massage and probing for and working out crystals. Engage with your partner so that you are well within their comfort level in the massage. If you have a partner that is ticklish, hold on to their feet without massaging until they relax. This may take several minutes. Children tend to be ticklish as well.

Children love foot massage. They love to be involved. At home, you can allow them to participate, at their own level of play. They do not have the concentration or hand strength of an adult. If they give you a one-minute foot massage, praise them for it. It can be a fun family event.

Natural oil, like almond oil or a natural massage lotion is best for the massage. The body will absorb anything that you put on your skin, so it is best to avoid petroleum based lotions and oils.

The amount of time you spend on foot massage is purely personal. Sometimes a few minutes are sufficient. In classes at the University we spend about twenty minutes per person. I know you will enjoy this technique and it is a valuable skill that will serve you, your family and friends in the years to come!

Foot Massage Chart

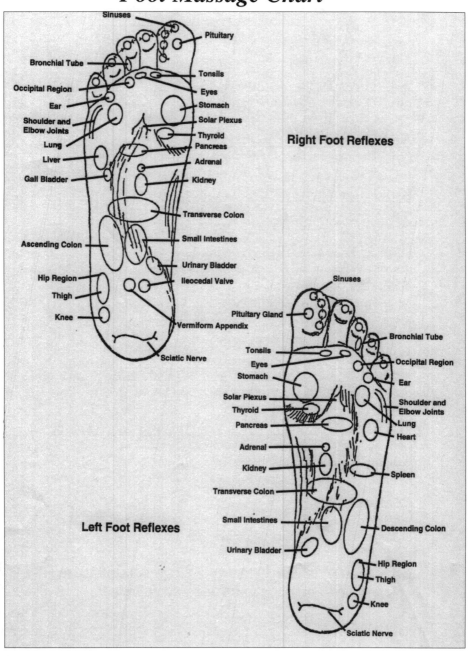

Suggested Reading And Viewing

VIDEOS

Kundalini Yoga: A Complete Course For Beginners
(six volumes) Nirvair Singh Khalsa, NSK Productions

Kundalini Yoga for Relaxation
Nirvair Singh Khalsa, NSK Productions

Kundalini Yoga For Relaxation II Runners And Skiers
Nirvair Singh Khalsa, NSK Productions

Heal Your Back Now!
(Book, video & CD) Nirvair Singh Khalsa,
NSK Productions
Morning Yoga Stretch/Evening Yoga Relaxation
Nirvair Singh Khalsa   NSK Productions

BOOKS

Kundalini Yoga-The Flow of Eternal Power
Shakti Parwha Kaur Khalsa Perigee Books

The Eight Human Talents: The Yogic Way to Restoring the
Natural Balance of Serenity Within You
Gurmukh Kaur Khalsa Harper Collins

Breathwalk
Gurucharan Singh Khalsa Broadway Books of Random
House

All videos & books by Nirvair Singh Khalsa are available online at http://www.KundaliniYoga.net